How To Lose Weight Fast

Unlocking the secrets of

effective weight loss

I0467179

Dr. Cara Slimming

Contents

CHAPTER ONE

Introduction to Acxion Fentermina

Fentermina is an over-the-counter weight loss drug manufactured by Acxion pharmaceuticals. It's an anorectic drug, meaning it suppresses appetite and helps people lose weight. Fentermina is made of fentermine hydroxide and it is available in both extended release and immediate release forms. Fentermina is indicated for short term use in the treatment of obesity for patience with a body mass index of 30 or greater. Fentermina works by stimulating the release of hormones in the brain that controls appetite. Specifically, Fentermina increases the levels of neropinephrine, serotine and dopamine which controls hunger and reduce food cravings. Fentermina also helps reduce the accumulation of fat by increasing the body's metabolism.

Possible Side Effects of Acxion Fentermina

Fentermina is a diet only pill used to treat obesity.It's used as an appetite suppressant to help reduce calorie intake and aid in weight loss. While Fentermina may be effective in helping people lose weight, it can also cause some unwanted side effects.

The most common side effects associated with Fentermina include: dry mouth, constipation, dizziness, insomnia and restlessness. These symptoms may be mild and temporary but they may become more severe and last longer. Other side effects include increased heart rate, increased blood pressure and increased risk of stroke. Long time use of Fentermina and also lead to an increased risk of dependence and addiction. More serious side effects associated with Fentermina can include an increase in anxiety, depression and suicidal thoughts. It's important to contact a doctor if you experience any of these serious side effects. Fentermina also has the potential to interact with certain medications such as antidepressants, blood thinners and seizure medications. It's important to tell your doctor about all medications you're taking before taking Acxion fentermina. Women who are pregnant or nursing should not use acxion fentermina. The drug has the potential to bring harm to an unborn baby or a nursing baby. It's also important to talk to your doctor if you are planning on becoming pregnant while taking Acxion Fentermina.

People with pre-existing conditions such heart disease, kidney disease, liver disease, should also talk to a doctor before taking Acxion fentermina. The drug can increase the risk of serious side effects in people with these conditions. Fentermina can also lead to dehydration. It's important to stay well dehydrated while taking Acxion fentermina, and to talk to doctor if you are experiencing any signs of dehydration such as dry mouth, dizziness and fatigue.

Benefits of Acxion Fentermina

Fentermina is a prescription weight loss medication designed to help people lose weight and improve their health. It's a stimulant type medication that works by increasing the activity of certain neurotransmitters in the brain. This increase in activity is thought to decrease appetite and increase energy both of which can help with weight loss. Fentermina has been used for decades in the USA and it is FDA approved for long term weight management. Fentermina has several benefits for those looking to lose weight. It can help reduce hunger, increase energy and boost metabolism. Fentermina can also help curb cravings which can make it easier to stick to a healthy. Additionally, it can help reduce food intake and make it easier to stick to a calorie controlled diet. Another benefit of Fentermina is that it can help improve mood and increase overall motivation. This can be beneficial for those who struggle with emotional issues related to weight loss. Fentermina can also help improve concentration and focus which can be beneficial for those who struggle to stay on track with a diet and exercise program.

Those Who Should Not Use Acxion Fentermina

Fentermina is a prescription only diet prescribed by doctors to help people lose weight. While it can be an effective tool for weight loss there are certain people who should not use it.First, Fentermina should not be used by people who have a history of heart disease. This drug can increase the risk of heart blood pressure, palpitation and other cardiac issues. It can also interact with certain heart medications so it should be used with caution. Secondly, Fentermina should not be used by people who have a history of drug abuse or addiction. This drug can be addictive and can cause severe withdrawal symptoms if the user stops taking it. It is important to be aware of the potential for abuse and addiction before taking Acxion fentermina. Fentermina should not be used by pregnant women or nursing mothers. This drug can pass into breast milk and cause negative effects on a developing baby. Fentermina should not be used by people who have a history of anxiety, depression and other mental issues. This drug can increase the risk of a maniac episode or other mental health problems so it should be avoided by those with a history of such issues.

CHAPTER TWO

Dose of Acxion Fentermina

Fentermina is a prescription weight loss medication that is used to help pwople with obesity lose weight. Fentermina is a sympathomimetic amine which is a type of drug that act on the sympathetic nervous system stimulating the release of certain hormones such as nonrepinephrine which can help suppress appetite. Fentermina is not approved by FDA for long term use and should only be used as part of a comprehensive weight loss program that includes diet, exercise and behavior modification. The recommended dosage for Fentermina is 15mg to 30mg taken orally once a day in the morning. The dose should be taken on an empty stomach at least one hour before breakfast. Patients should also drink plenty of fluids throughout the day to help prevent dehydration. It is important to follow the instruction on the product label and to consult with a healthcare professional before taking or adjusting the dosage.

Alternatives to Acxion fentermina

The most common alternative to Fentermina is lifestyle changes; this includes engaging in a healthy diet and regular physical activity. Making these changes is often the best way to achieve everlasting weight loss and improved health. Diet and exercise are natural, safe and cost effective. Another alternative to Fentermina is using other prescription medication such as orlistat. However, they can also have potential side effect so it is important to talk to your doctor about the risk and benefits of these medications. There are also non-prescription alternatives to Acxion fentermina, which includes natural supplement such as garcinia, cambogia, green tea extract, and caffeine. While these supplements have been used for weight loss they have not be proven to be as effective as prescription medications.

How should Fentermina be taken

It's important to take it responsibly in order to maximize its benefits and minimize its potential risk. While taking acxion fentermina, it's important to follow the directions on the label and to only take the prescribed dosage. Taking more than the recommended dosage can increase the risk of side effects such as insomnia, dizziness, heart palpitations. It's also important to take Fentermina with a full glass of water as this helps to ensure that it is absorbed quickly and efficiently. It's important to take Fentermina same time each day as this helps to ensure that the medication remains at constant levels in the body. It's also important to take Fentermina with a meal or snacks as this helps to reduce the risk of side effects. It is important to know that Fentermina may interact with certain medications such as antidepressant, so it's important to discuss any potential interactions with your doctor before taking Acxion fentermina. It's also important to keep in mind that Fentermina may cause withdrawal symptoms if it's suddenly stopped, so it's important to avoid abruptly stopping the medication. If you need to stop taking Acxion fentermina, it's important to do so gradually under the direction of your doctor.

Precautions

The first precaution to take while using Fentermina is to follow the dosage instructions provided by your doctor. It's important to take the medications exactly as prescribed in order to avoid serious side effects. Fentermina should be taken on an empty stomach at least one hour before meals. If you are taking other medications then you should check with your doctor to ensure that the two medications do not interact negatively.

Secondly, you should be aware of the potential side effects of Acxion fentermina. Common side effects may include: insomnia, dizziness, dry mouth, headaches, constipation, and anxiety. If you experience any of these side effects, stop taking your medication and talk to your doctor right away.

Storage Instructions of Acxion Fentermina

Fentermina is usually taken once a day and should be stored in a safe place at room temperature. When storing Acxion fentermina, it's important to keep the medication in its original container and store it at room temperature. It should not be exposed to excessive heat, cold or moisture. The medication is also sensitive to light so it should be stored in a dark dry place.

When to see a doctor

While Fentermina can help people lose weight, it should not be used without medical supervision. Before taking Acxion fentermina, it's important to consult with a doctor to discuss potential risks and benefits. This includes if you have any preexisting medical conditions such as high blood pressure, diabetes, liver or kidney disease as well as if you have any other medication or supplement already being taken. A doctor will also be able to access your overall health and determine if Fentermina is the right weight loss solution for you. It's important to see

a doctor while taking Acxion
fentermina.

THE END